THE
MANSFORMATION
DIET

MITCH CALVERT

Disclaimer:

(1) Introduction This disclaimer governs the use of this book. [By using this book, you accept this disclaimer in full. / We will ask you to agree to this disclaimer before you can access the book.]

No part of this book may be reproduced in any written, electronic, recording, or photocopying without written permission of the author. All trademarks are the exclusive property of mitchcalvert.com

(2) Credit

This disclaimer was created using an SEQ Legal template.

(3) No advice The book contains information about men's dieting from the perspective of the author. The information is not advice, and should not be treated as such. You must not rely on the information in the book as an alternative to medical advice from an appropriately qualified professional. If you have any specific questions about any matter you should consult an appropriately qualified medical professional. If you think you may be suffering from any medical condition you should seek immediate medical attention. You should never delay seeking medical advice, disregard medical advice, or discontinue medical treatment because of information in this book

(4) No representations or warranties

To the maximum extent permitted by applicable law and subject to section 6 below, we exclude all representations, warranties, undertakings and guarantees relating to the book. Without prejudice to the generality of the foregoing paragraph, we do not represent, warrant, undertake or guarantee:

- that the information in the book is correct, accurate, complete or non-misleading;

- that the use of the guidance in the book will lead to any particular outcome or result;

(5) Limitations and exclusions of liability

The limitations and exclusions of liability set out in this section and elsewhere in this disclaimer: are subject to section 6 below; and govern all liabilities arising under the disclaimer or in relation to the book, including liabilities arising in contract, in tort (including negligence) and for breach of statutory duty. We will not be liable to you in respect of any losses arising out of any event or events beyond our reasonable control. We will not be liable to you in respect of any business losses, including without limitation loss of or damage to profits, income, revenue, use, production, anticipated savings, business, contracts, commercial opportunities or goodwill. We will not be liable to you in respect of any loss or corruption of any data, database or software. We will not be liable to you in respect of any special, indirect or consequential loss or damage.

(6) Exceptions

Nothing in this disclaimer shall: limit or exclude our liability for death or personal injury resulting from negligence; limit or exclude our liability for fraud or fraudulent misrepresentation; limit any of our liabilities in any way that is not permitted under applicable law; or exclude any of our liabilities that may not be excluded under applicable law.

(7) Severability

If a section of this disclaimer is determined by any court or other competent authority to be unlawful and/or unenforceable, the other sections of this disclaimer continue in effect. If any unlawful and/or unenforceable section would be lawful or enforceable if part of it were deleted, that part will be deemed to be deleted, and the rest of the section will continue in effect.

(8) Our details In this disclaimer, "we" means (and "us" and "our" refer to) Mitch Calvert (Manitoba, Canada) and team and or any future addresses, temporary or permanent."

Table of Contents

About the Author

Mitch is a transformation coach for men like his former self, with worse genes than Chris Farley. Yes, the heavy-set chap from Tommy Boy who was goddamn hilarious but died too young.

Wanna hear more from him? Go to www.mitchcalvert.com. You'll find hundreds of articles on all things men's fitness. You'll also be presented the opportunity to enjoy a steady stream of "Mitch-ism" emails. All designed to help you build your best body.

FREE Download: Have a fair bit of fat to lose, especially in the belly? Need a place to start in 30 seconds or less? Grab this easily digestible (pun intended) two-page cheat sheet for men, to simplify your diet without fads, quick fixes or calorie counting, courtesy of coach Mitch, free for Mansformation Diet readers.

Is the Mansformation Diet right for?

Any diet-strategy has to become a lifestyle if it's going to lead to permanent results. It's an effective motivator to have short-term goals, but without a permanent plan you will gain back all the weight. Yo-Yo dieting like this hurts your metabolism and psyche, sometimes irrevocably. Don't be a Jonah Hill.

All diets require true dedication if you are going to be successful with them. But after decades in the business, having coached hundreds to successful transformations, this is the most sustainable plan I've found that allows for balance.

My gym teacher called me fat

I haven't always been a fitness coach, a columnist with AskMen and lived this lifestyle.

It was in gym class back in 2002, and the Omron body fat tester told me everything I already knew – I was fat. The reading came up at 35.5% body fat – the worst score among the guys in the class.

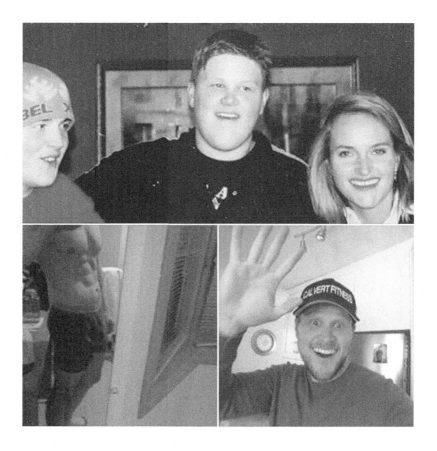

That moment told me I needed to change, but I didn't actually do anything at first.

That was until my brother Caleb came home with a massive bag of protein powder and Arnold Schwarzenegger's Pumping Iron on DVD.

Knowing my younger brother was getting in shape inspired me to do the same. I told myself if I didn't follow suit, I'd have to quit playing video games for a year (a BIG deal to me at the time) and wrote a sticky note on my computer monitor to blackmail myself to stick to it.

But here's the lesson for you: don't see your weight loss goal as something you can achieve in 30 or 60 days and then go back to your old habits.

In my time, I've had some EPIC failures in my own fat loss journey. Name a mistake and I've probably made it over the past 14 years since losing 60 pounds.

I wasted time on workout programs that didn't work.

I've wasted money on BS supplements.

And I even ended up in the emergency room of a hospital after following an extreme fad diet for too long.

Seriously, the number of times I've been left embarrassed and out of pocket with nothing to show for it...

You name a mistake, I've probably done it.

Still, my loss is your gain, and the key thing is that I've LEARNED from my mistakes.

I want to make sure you don't fall for the same faux pas I did, so read on.

Fat Loss Secrets Revealed

I lived like a monk in pursuit of the perfect body for years.

I watched everything I put in my mouth and sacrificed a lot.

I would never eat the foods I loved — and never dared miss a meal for fear of losing 'muscle'

On top of that, I trained excessively as often as I could.

Did it work?

Sure, but I could've gotten there an easier way.

Let me explain...

These days, I only get to the gym four times a week if I'm lucky. I'm coaching hundreds of guys to their own transformations, have a beautiful family and work with guys across the globe.

I eat cinnamon buns, hamburgers and fries, and ice cream and guess what?

I found a way to look and feel great anyway.

In this book, I'm going to reveal a secret almost ALL of the "experts" don't share.

One that can GREATLY accelerate your fat loss progress.

It's probably the exact opposite of what you've been told to do to lose body fat.

The good news? It's brain-dead simple to do and you're going to love it.

Even BETTER news? You get to eat all kinds of DELICIOUS foods you were probably told were taboo.

Ready for the secret? To lose body fat you need to... EAT LESS FOOD THAN YOU NEED TO MAINTAIN YOUR WEIGHT!

That's right.

But you want to do it while enjoying life, right?

After spending a few years perfecting the eating strategy, I finally put it all into a program you need to live a life free of Tupperware, be comfortable going shirtless at the pool, while still achieving new goals in the gym.

And it's all in this book you're reading.

The Dreaded Man Boobs

Gold's Gym was the reason I started lifting weights in the first place.

I was 260 pounds and addicted to video games at the time, and watching the documentary, Pumping Iron, where many scenes were filmed in Gold's Venice, got me out of the funk and into the gym for the first time.

In fact, this has me going back down memory lane...

I remember always wearing two shirts back then, so my moobs (man boobs) would be hidden. No tight shirts or white shirts. Maybe you could relate at one time or still do?

I developed a really poor posture to hide from the world further, shoulders hunched over.

This is one of the reasons I make it my mission to help men transform their bodies and lives. Because I know how it feels.

I still get a little weird taking my shirt off, because I remember avoiding those social events like the plague.

Shirts vs. skins basketball? I'm out.

Pool party? No chance.

Living with that shame isn't fun. But even more tragic are the joys of life one misses.

And 'moobs' are a tell tale sign your hormonal environment is skewed the wrong way as a man (estrogen up, test down). Nothing is worse for your hormones than being above 20% bodyfat.

In fact, one study shows a significant drop in testosterone the heavier you get, greatly increasing your risk of death, let alone everyday discomforts.

They Laughed At Me

"Oh, no."

That was my thought as I struggled to move the barbell. I wondered if this was the end of my short tenure into the gym.

Those are the thoughts that race through your head when you lay trapped beneath your own bench press; the cold iron grazing your throat.

Thankfully, a far more experienced gym goer came over and saved me from my embarrassment.

I'm not sure how I thought I could bench 185 lbs in my second week EVER in the gym.

Hell, it had been hard enough to convince myself I'd be welcome there. Growing up I was overweight. OK, more than just an above average chubby kid – I was obese. Which is OK for some, but I was self-conscious about it and the target of jokes in high school.

I wanted to be isolated because I was embarrassed. And I was able to avoid things by hiding in plain sight. I wanted my gym visits to be the same.

I used to think they were talking about me every time I saw someone laugh...

"Do you see that guy?" somebody chuckled.

The others around him laughed...

At least that was the reality I had built in my head.

But I carried on.

Because the gym doesn't allow for hiding.

And it changed my life.

Now there is no laughter, but rather respect.

The same kids in high school who laughed at me are now sporting dad bods and Facebook messaging me for advice.

"Where did you learn?" . . . "How long have you trained?" . . . "What do you eat and when?" "Must have a FAST metabolism (lol)"

I hold no ill-will towards them. They probably didn't even realize the impact their teasing had on me. In fact, I should thank them.

It forced me to change.

Are YOU hiding from something?

All of us are.

Hiding from change. Hiding from responsibility. Hiding from the prospect of feeling foolish.

We hide by avoiding things that will change us. We hide by letting someone else speak up and lead and get the girls and get the good jobs and get the life satisfaction.

We will rationalize in extraordinary ways to avoid coming out of hiding.

But I don't hide very often these days. And the process of getting in shape – venturing into that gym for the first time – set the stage for that confidence.

Over 15 years later, after helping guys and girls like my former self overcome the same barriers and get in great shape themselves, I still remember how my strength was sparked by that first failure on the bench press.

There were countless other failures that followed, but they've all helped shape the man I am today (figuratively and physically)

Hopefully you'll use the turning of the calendar to step up and answer the call. And to open your eyes and see that you can have the life you want. If you are prepared to work for it.

Your story is sabotaging you

I don't have the genetics to have a six-pack abs. I don't like vegetables enough to eat clean. I don't have the time to cook the kinds of foods that I need to be eating.

Those were the thoughts I struggled with. It's not until I frankly called bullshit on it all, and focused instead on enjoying the process instead of the elusive final result, that I turned the corner for good.

You talk to yourself in a way that you would never allow anyone else to speak to you. You are harsh on yourself. You are mean-spirited. You are cynical. Most of us are.

But if you concentrate on stopping that negative self-talk, you start to reprogram your unconscious. You start to change the way you think. It really is that simple. It doesn't happen in a day, but it truly is that simple.

"The hardest thing to understand is just how easy it is to change it all."

When you figure out the voice in your head is just replaying a story you've created, you can then take control of those thoughts and banish them for good.

I'm reading a book these days by Carol Dweck, which outlines two types of mindsets.

You either have a fixed or growth mindset to varying degrees – but you CAN change.

Growth mindsets tend to learn from criticism rather than ignoring it, overcome challenges rather than avoiding them, and find inspiration in the success of others rather than feeling threatened.

A fixed mindset is quite the opposite – you think you're doomed to the skill set you have currently, whether it's in a sport, regarding your intelligence, or your body type. But none of those things are fixed – the research Dweck points to proves that out.

"Gifted" kids with a fixed mindset hold themselves back, while "average" kids with growth mindsets achieve great things because they aren't afraid to fail and go after the things they want. The same with adults. It's never too late. A fixed mindset was something I battled with for years – and it still holds me back in some areas of my life.

So this isn't a cakewalk to overcome.

But changing your mindset needs to be one of the first things you work on. You could be given the BEST diet and exercise plan in the world, but if it's planted in a fixed mindset, the likelihood of success is slim to none.

My clients who get these massive transformations are not miraculously waking up with a new body.

They focus on the process. They focus on showing up to train, even on days where they'd have a valid excuse not to. They focus on sticking to the schedule and "not quitting" even when the going gets tough or the scale indicates a bad week.

Then, one day, they realize the scale is down 50 lbs and they feel like a new person. But, again, it was a belief in the process that got them there. Not a narrow focus on the end result, but a growth mindset willing to overcome every challenge along the way.

Instead of worrying about getting six pack abs, commit to the process of eating healthy each day. Instead of worrying about buying that big house, commit to the process of earning more money each day. Instead of worrying, start doing through small daily actions.

This stuff is not limited to fitness by any means. Mindset. Is. Everything.

How Do You Shift to a Growth Mindset?

I'm not big on writing down goals, New Year's resolutions, or gimmicky self-help gurus. But one way to truly see how your mind is helping or hindering you is to sit down for a few minutes each day and just write down whatever it is you're thinking. Full credit to Brian Grasso for turning me onto this simple – yet effective – strategy.

This serves a valuable purpose, because until you call awareness to what you are thinking, you often don't know what you're thinking. Silly, I know.

Grasso suggests, 9 times out of 10, when you do this journaling exercise a few times a day for at least a week or two, you're going to see some patterns.

"I feel tired. Lethargic. I have to go to the gym in a couple hours, but I don't feel like it. I don't want to go. I can't eat a good lunch. I'm too busy. I'm not good enough."

Those are the repeat thoughts you may be having over and over and over again all day long, and you're not even aware you're having them. That's the stuff that needs to be cut loose in order to be successful – in whatever pursuit you're after.

You have to shift your thoughts – and truly start to enjoy the process of getting in shape, as without some level of enjoyment in the journey, the destination will never be within reach.

Remember those past diets that helped you lose weight fast? They were built on an unrealistic level of willpower. You hated every minute of it, which is why you fell off and rebounded back to your starting weight.

I know it's unfair... the harder you focus on your weight loss goal, the less likely it's to come. Just like the more you focus on getting that new car or promotion, the less likely it's to come. Instead, focus on the process. The action steps needed to move closer to your goal, and put in the work. That's where the secret sauce is.

Lessons from Shia LaBeouf

Full disclosure: I own an "Enough LaBeouf" t-shirt. But that purchase preceded this video where tells us to "JUST DO IT", which changed my perspective on him. I only wear that t-shirt to bed nowadays out of pure shame.

The biggest lesson here... is the 'compound effect'

Do something daily to move you forward.

Every

Single

Day

Do

Something

When it comes to fitness, get a good sweat going every day.

If you aren't forced to change clothes at least once, it was a day lost.

Your body is programmed to move, a lot, so don't let modern life ruin that for you. Get going.

Is that a chicken breast in your pocket or are you just happy to see me?

It was a sunny June afternoon circa 2009 and I was heading to a UFC event with a few buddies.

We got there early to take in the festivities, and I figured I would go for at least six hours without a proper meal.

So, naturally, I packed a chicken breast smothered with peanut butter in my pocket.

Unfortunately, the bouncer at the door frisked me, found the chicken breast, and inquired, "WTF is that?" I explained my predicament — and the muscle loss that would surely follow — and he said I was mostly at risk for salmonella and suggested I eat it right then and there or he'd toss it out.

Long story short, I had to force down some dry chicken in front of a line-up of UFC fans. Hardcore.

So what am I trying to tell you with this trip down memory lane?

In the early days of my fitness journey as a young and naive Mitch, I replaced one obsession (junk food and video games) with another (extreme weight lifting and healthy eating) instead of taking a balanced approach.

I withdrew myself further from the world, measuring every morsel of food that went into my mouth, refusing to eat dinner with my family and avoiding social gatherings so I could maximize my deep sleep.

It took a while to come to the realization that I was wasting some of the best years of my life to try to maximize my results in the gym.

My approach now focuses on balance and moderation (in fact, I get better results now that I've loosened the reins a bit) and that's ultimately what my clients want, too. (If you need help finding a middle-of-the-road approach that works, check out this <u>free fat loss cheat sheet for men</u>.)

So I want to let you know that you can reach your fat loss goals while enjoying barbecues and beers. Here's how.

It's All Bullshit

If you're new to the fitness industry, you're in trouble. Plain and simple. There are thousands of fat cats in the tall grass waiting to gnaw on your cute, little mouse ears. Tread with caution or get eaten alive by fitness industry scams.

You must be thinking *"Are you on pain meds and delirious, Mitch? What's this cat and mouse analogy you speak of?"* Sorry, it's the best I can do, and I'm drug-free at the moment. Maybe I'd come up with something better if I was looped right now, but I know for sure I'd resort to stiff drugs if I had to endure what you're about to if starting a healthy lifestyle is on your list of resolutions.

A noble cause to be sure, but sadly you're in for a world of hurt. You logically start your search on Google and instantly get confused. One site tells you to eat carbs. Another says to avoid them entirely and just eat fats. Eat gluten. Don't eat gluten. Only buy organic vegetables harvested in the far northern plains of the Shire. Buy soy. Oh, wait, no, avoid soy, it'll give you man boobs.

"Is that only 85% cocao dark chocolate? Dude, that's not going to improve your heart health. Eat this rock-hard square of 99% cacao, it tastes like cardboard, and you'll have to sit it on your tongue for a half hour to absorb the bitterness, but it sure works! My heart has never been stronger" – Signed, Crossfit-Paleo-Caveman Warrior.

You end up leaving the Google search exercise more confused than ever. And it's not your fault. There is so much information available at your fingertips, that trimming the fat and separating the useful from the useless is an impossible task.

The fitness industry loves extremes – going to the extremes sells really well. But try being honest, telling people it'll be at least 16 weeks of dedicated eating and training before they'll see any drastic changes, and they'll head somewhere else.

This is a lifestyle you need to buy into long-term to see results. If you don't make a habit of it, the weight loss will revert to weight gain as soon as your motivation falls off.

Secret revealed: Most contestants on NBC's "The Biggest Loser" gain back a lot of the weight they lose on the show within a year or so, a fact that one of the show's former trainers, Jillian Michaels, admitted to The Nashville Tennessean news agency.

Working out for five or six hours a day – day after day – leads to drastic weight loss, and that makes for good TV, but it's clearly not sustainable. Just like dropping your calories to less than 1,000 a day will do the same, but nor is it sustainable.

"Fat is good and carbs are bad? Cool, let me guzzle mayo by the gallon and lather my bacon with pounds of butter every morning. I'll then wash it down with a coffee blended with 6 cups of butter and 14 tablespoons of MCT (coconut) oil. I'm in a fat burning zone!" – Signed, "Bulletproof" Coffee Guru

No, sorry, bud. Your calories are ridiculously high (fat has 9 calories per gram!) in relation to your daily expenditure, and eating fat to those extremes is neither good for you, or part of a healthy, balanced diet.

And that's really the point here. **Moderation is not such a bad thing.** Permanently banning foods from your diet is going to make you crave them even more. Do you know why your little one loves candy so much? Because you make it desirable for them by limiting it. The law of scarcity in full view.

You shouldn't bar yourself from the odd treat (hell, eat a pizza dipped in ice cream one night if it suits your fancy) unless you've got a legitimate allergy or are the type who can finish an entire jar of peanut butter in one sitting.

If that's the case, don't keep the temptations in the house. Curse you, Costco-sized Boom Chicka Pop, by the way. Your deceptively low-calorie count justifies binging.

The 30,000 Foot Epiphany

I was flying to LA for a conference.

Since there's no direct flights from Winnipeg, I spent a fair bit of time in planes and automobiles (no trains, though it would've helped with the wording of this sentence).

I was on a flight between Minneapolis and Winnipeg on the way home.

A guy sits down beside me. We exchange some small talk, and then come to realize we both have a daughter around the same age. He looked well north of 40. Protruding belly. Puffy face. Bags under his eyes.

You could tell he wasn't comfortable in his own skin. Kept pulling at his shirt and trying to huddle smaller in his chair as to not infringe on my personal space.

I wanted to tell him "hey, I've been there" and not to sweat it, but didn't have the balls to say it.

Heck, I was the dude wearing a shirt in the pool not too long ago, 50 pounds overweight.

And now that the shoe is on the other foot, it's easy to forget.

I quietly observed his food choices and could've given him some tips right then and there. But that's not my style nor appropriate IMO.

If I did, I would recommend he bring beef jerky and a water on the plane rather than ordering a snack pack loaded with calories and two rye and cokes (as he did on the hour-long flight).

After talking about what we do for a living, this guy looks at me and says, "I'm sick and tired of being sick and tired. I want to be a role model for my daughter, but I don't know where to start"

A light bulb went off right then and there.

How can guys who feel overwhelmed by life regain their former glory without living in the gym?

I'm not talking about a fad diet that leads to some initial weight loss but tanks your metabolism.

I'm not talking about some hardcore fitness model routine that leaves you broken at the end.

I'm talking about turning your dad bod into something you can be proud of with the minimum effective dose of exercise and dieting.

For some reason, as you age you "accept" the way things are.

Your beer gut or muffin top. Your lack of energy and vitality. Your diminished sex drive.Your dreaded man boobs.

Yes, getting older come with more stress and responsibility, and less time for the gym.

You end up with a Bowflex masquerading as a clothes hanger and a Hummer-sized spare tire. But it doesn't have to be all or nothing.

It takes work to change deeply ingrained habits, I get that.

But it's usually a lot easier than you think.

Maybe you're fine with how you look and feel. There's no mandatory requirement that you need to look a certain way.

But if it's affecting your happiness…

Your job prospects…

Your family life…

Your mood…

You owe it to yourself to start making a change.

The future you doesn't like you

Do you ever stay up too late watching Netflix and curse yourself when the alarm goes off the next morning?

It's a far too common problem I see clients make.

You know a lack of sleep is correlated with bad stuff (yes, that's the scientific term)

But seem unable to see the big picture in the moment.

While watching the Netflix documentary *Jerry Before Seinfeld* past my bedtime last night (oops), he addressed this failure of adulthood.

(Paraphrasing Jerry's words)

"I'm Night Guy. I stay up as late as I want.

Just one more episode, another sleeve of Oreos

'What about getting up after five hours sleep?' Oh, that's Morning Guy's problem. That's not my problem.

...Then you get up in the morning, the alarm rings, you're exhausted, groggy... Oh, I hate that Night Guy!

See, Night Guy always screws Morning Guy. There's nothing Morning Guy can do."

Research shows that when we think about ourselves in the future, it's like we're thinking about another person.

So Night Guy goes out drinking with his friends and Morning Guy gets stuck with the hangover.

There's Hungry Guy who leaves Fat Guy with a beer gut, Young Guy who doesn't save enough money for Old Guy to retire and so on.

Reframe How You See Yourself In The Moment

So, what can you do to avoid self-sabotage? How do you see the big picture, able to put off immediate gratification to get more sleep, eat better and exercise when that devil on your shoulder is telling you to do the opposite?

Researchers suggest you can change your thinking on this by introducing yourself...to your future self.

One clever way they have done this is to show people pictures of themselves that have been digitally aged.

If you're looking to lose weight, use pictures of yourself digitally fattened up and refer to that mental image in the moment.

When you see older or fatter versions of yourself, you are more likely to see your current and future self as the same person.

As the researchers said, "these types of interventions help people realize that their future selves are ultimately dependent on the choices that they make today."

What Richard Simmons can teach you about fat loss

I was wrong.

When I first became a coach, I thought every client would instantly buy in and find the passion for exercise and health to the same level I was at.

"OMG, is that purple kale from Australia? AWESOME!"

But, frankly, I was the weird one.

Because I completely forgot where I came from.

13 years ago, the gym was this foreign meat market with wall to ceiling windows and ripped dudes and hot chicks.

A diet was something Richard Simmons and hippies preached about (OK, I'm not that old) and certainly nothing I wanted to get myself into.

I was scared to go to the gym.

I was scared to face reality.

I was scared to get my shit handled because change is hard and my comfort zone was safe.

And there was good reason for that. This is NOT easy.

In fact, the first 6-12 months will be a terrible grind, especially if you're starting from ground zero.

But if you break through and come out on the other side? Awesomeness ensues, I promise you that.

Higher metabolic rate, more energy and confidence, little black dresses, Borat speedos, all while living a lifestyle with fitness as just ONE component. 4% of your day.

I have this client, we'll call him Trist (because it rhymes with his real name) who's been working with me for a couple months.

He's made a ton of progress, seems to have the healthy eating part down, is reading nutritional labels and preparing quality food, has lost weight, but is frustrated that he can't consistently get in the gym on his own when we aren't scheduled for in-person workouts.

But that's OK!

Going from 0-60 MPH out of the gates is not realistic. 0-20 after a month? Good. That's progress.

You'll get results from the minimum effective dose in the early going. So build one good habit at a time and see the long-term vision for yourself to keep you focused and on track.

I've had enough clients to know this by now. Not everyone comes to me at 60 MPH ready for purple Kale and cluster sets – some are just at the starting line or in the middle of the race going in circles.

That's why there's no one size fits all program. Nor is it just about getting lean so you have before/after pictures to show off (only to balloon up to your starting weight when you start eating again).

My programs never eliminate whole nutrient groups like carbs, fats, dairy or (GASP) gluten. My programs are setup to optimize hormonal and overall health, avoiding starvation and rebound dieting. My programs provide weight training plans that work for you, whether you like the gym or prefer the confines of your own home. Yes, you're going to have to sweat at some point.

It's not sexy, nor does it satisfy a need for instant gratification, but it flat out gets the job done.

Back row at your own funeral

It's wise to 'picture the end' sometimes...

What do I mean by that?

Well, envision yourself in the future.

One clever way researchers have done this is to show people pictures of themselves digitally aged.

If you're looking to lose weight, use pictures of yourself digitally fattened up and refer to that mental image in the moment.

When you see older or fatter versions of yourself, you are more likely to see your current and future self as the same person.

When you understand that your choices today shape your future – good or bad – you become self-aware.

Take it a step further and picture yourself at your OWN funeral.

Yikes. Uncomfortable.

But here's what this looks like...

Back Row At His Own Funeral

Someone you don't recognize is handing out programs, printed with the face of a white-haired guy in a suit.

Family members are taking the pews, which are otherwise bare.

You recognize the church, all cavernous and bare, and knew you'd be invisible in the back row.

They sure picked a shitty picture, you think, scanning the program.

You look fat.

"Couldn't they have found one with me smiling?"

But you knew the answer to that question.

You see your daughter and her newborn baby in the front row.

Her head is in her hands, crying.

You flashback to a special moment:

"Daddy, Daddy, Daddy! Come here, Daddy"

As she runs into the room, excited to share one of her projects from school.

Your eyes light up at the thought.

But just as instantly, you feel a sense of deep regret in the pit of your stomach.

"You knew at that moment, didn't you, asshole?"

Your bad habits were slowly leading you down this path...

"So why didn't you get off the couch?"

Fuck.

Your wife is across the aisle.

Boy, she looks like she's aged 10 years since you last locked eyes on her.

More people drift through now, a cell phone goes off, and you see your brother reach for a tissue.

This is it.

You'll be leaving this room in an urn, a tidy departure from this world.

Left to collect dust on a shelf.

But better than rotting six feet under, you figure.

At least that was your thought process when arrangements were made and the will was written.

Your brother takes the stand.

He talks about all the usual BS spewed at these things: you were a good father, husband, hard-working man.

He throws in a few stories that bring about a stifled laugh or two from friends.

You drift off and are overcome by a memory of the two of you and your dad.

"Dad, your head looks like an egg," you said in front of the whole team of bantam hockey players, prompting shocked, amused laughter from teammates.

He was just blasting us for a bad period of play, too.

Dad eventually went full Bruce Willis and kept it shaved down to the bone – no more bald spot.

Still looked like an egg...

Now it's your aunt's turn to speak.

What's she got to say?

More of the usual stuff. Boring.

Watching your relatives step up, overcome by emotion, triggers another memory.

It was a summer day like any other.

You were stocking shelves at the local Safeway and that dick head manager of yours flags you down, talking on the phone like he'd seen a ghost.

Not the usual high-and-mighty smirk you were used to seeing when he came to bark orders at you.

Odd, you thought.

"Your mom is on the phone," manager Dick Head says.

You were just 16 when your father died suddenly of a heart attack.

You showed no emotion on that phone call or at the funeral.

Kept it all bottled up inside.

Family members reacted with awkward, stiff sympathies, leaving you confused and guilty for not crying.

What did they want?

You felt a loss – for sure – but how did they expect you to express any of it at that age?

You should've vowed to take care of yourself, you think...

The genetic lottery was working against you. Your dad's sudden death was proof of that.

At this point, the minister seems to look right at you: "The floor's open, if anyone wishes to speak."

You jump to attention.

Of course, you'd like to...

Tell everyone how thankful you are.

Tell everyone how much you're going to miss them.

Tell everyone how much you wish you could've stopped drinking and eating yourself to an early grave.

But it's too late.

Your story has been written.

No do-overs.

Chapter 1

What to do when you've tried it all

You've probably tried everything when it comes to fitness.

1) Eat less, move more

2) Do cardio (fasted OMG!!)

3) Detox

4) Join a Crossfit gym

5) Amputate a limb

... Right?

And some of it is OK advice. If you can stick to it.

But here's the thing:

For every guru sayin' this is all it takes...

... you've got, what, like millions of people who got nowhere trying any or all of it?

We do have an obesity epidemic after all.

So what gives?

I'll tell ya...

The difference between those who make it and those who fail, rinse and repeat...

Usually comes down to one of 4 things:

1) Information overload. There's too much info consumption, not enough action.

2) No wiggle room. Your diet will fail without room for failure, if you feel me?

3) Eating wrong for your genetics. Find the right diet for your genetic blueprint, not that juiced up bodybuilder's plan.

4) Accountability. If it's only you in the fight, I promise your brain will sabotage you at every turn.

Any of that sound familiar?

If so, I'm glad you're reading this.

I help average people simplify fitness and get results.

Just what you need, right?

… Another guy claiming his approach to fitness is the ONLY way.

Look, I get it.

You need another diet strategy like I need a swift kick to the gonads.

(Not very badly.)

Lucky for you, I don't have one.

What I do have, however, is a smarter, simpler, speedier approach to getting the results you want… even if you've tried it all in the past.

And since there's zero chance you believe me, how 'bout I just show you?

Keep reading.

How Spud Lost 60 Pounds Without Eating One Potato

"You know, Spud, what happened to you?"

"You used to be the most in shape guy in here, and now you're just a fat fuck."

Sure, the guy was drunk. But hearing that stung. Sometimes the nectar of the Gods can be a truth serum, and that night at the bar was a turning point.

Like being smashed in the face with a stack of bricks, Spud had his weight loss wake-up call.

That defining moment where you realize the pain of staying the same is greater than the pain of change.

And with that, he'd had enough.

He joined my Mansformation 2.0 program on the recommendation of a friend, David, who had lost 40 pounds going through it himself and the rest, as cliché as it sounds, is history, as you'll read about below.

But let's back up a bit here first.

"Spud" was always the bigger kid growing up.

That's how he earned the nickname, in fact.

Back in the third grade, he called his skinny friend "Green Bean" [his last name Green plus his likeness to string beans), and, in retaliation, Green Bean called him Spud because of his resemblance to a potato.

Anyway, there's the context here, but we're getting sidetracked.

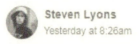

Steven Lyons
Yesterday at 8:26am

Month 9. Never felt better. Thanks Coach! The key for me, patience.

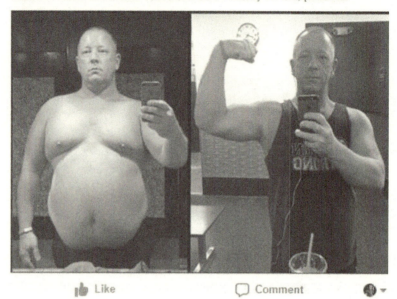

👍 Like   💬 Comment   ⚫ ▾

But you want to know how Spud was able to lose so much weight, right?

Starvation? Amputation? Green coffee bean extract?

No, thankfully, none of that.

Simple math, really.

SPUD FOCUSED ON CALORIES

According to a review on Examine.com, when it comes to weight loss, the most important factor is eating less.

"Independent of your diet's macronutrient ratios, a negative energy balance (consuming fewer calories than your body needs) is responsible for weight loss."

Basically, Spud stopped eating so much crap.

But, unlike previous attempts, he didn't resort to starving himself with a steady diet of celery sticks and ice cubes.

He gave his body everything it needed through balanced meals with an emphasis on protein.

IT'S NOT ALL OR NOTHING

For the vast majority of people, as long as your calories stay in a deficit—there is zero reason you can't also enjoy some "off plan" foods.

Flexible dieting sometimes gets a bad rap because people assume it means eating nothing but doughnuts, cake, and brownies.

But, in Spud's case, he got rid of the junk in his fridge and focused primarily on healthy, balanced meals, with the odd controlled cheat thrown in.

HABITS OVER MOTIVATION

Spud then focused on habits.

He upped his step count (off days spent at the beach) and commitment to the gym, scheduling in workouts like job appointments.

Habits are the key.

Ever notice that when you start a new endeavour, you're incredibly motivated?

But when that motivation fizzles... you jump ship, right?

Every blogger starts incredibly motivated.

However, after one or two posts that no one has read, shared, or commented on— the passion fades.

Think those people would quit if their first blog post had a million views and 600 comments?

The same thing happens with your diet.

But, here's the thing.

KEEP GOING

Once the "positive feedback loop" of your efforts shows up, nothing can stop you.

Spud works in a bar.

He sees the same people day after day, and now that he's losing weight by the day, the compliments are coming in fast and furious.

That positive feedback reinforces his efforts. It's human nature.

Weight loss is challenging— expect motivation to abandon you during the grind but return once the positive feedback of what you're doing comes in waves.

THINK BEYOND WEIGHT LOSS

For Spud, the weight and belly fat losses have been secondary to his improved mental state.

"Losing weight is awesome, and I'm hearing it from people every day now. Total validation. But the number one thing for me is my head," Spud says. "My head is different now. When you suffer from anxiety and depression, and you're carrying around 274 pounds, you can't win.

"My ability to handle my anxiety is much more in control now because my head is clear and I have good things in my body. The people that normally try to push my buttons can't find them anymore," he adds.

Your metabolism doesn't suck (most likely)

If you're stuck trying to lose a few lbs you're not alone.

I speak to dozens of guys every day who send me messages telling me things aren't working anymore.

"I'm stuck at this weight no matter what I do"

"I used to always be able to follow this diet for awhile and drop 10 lbs but it doesn't work anymore..."

"I can't gain an ounce of muscle no matter what I try, and my spare tire isn't going anywhere, either"

You see, your body is programmed to keep you alive. It does a good job of that, but it can be a big pain in the arse when dieting.

When you try to outsmart your body, it outsmarts you back.

If you try to rush the process, here's how your body tries to keep your weight steady when you take in less energy and start to lose weight, according to Precision Nutrition...

- **Thermic effect of food** goes down because you're eating less.

- **Resting metabolic rate** goes down because you weigh less.

- Calories burned through **physical activity** go down.

- **Non-exercise activity thermogenesis** goes down.

- **Calories not absorbed** goes down and you absorb more of what you eat because your body senses a calorie deficit.

- Reducing actual calories eaten also causes **hunger signals** to increase, causing you to crave (and maybe eat) more.

Definitions of each below

Thermic effect of food (TEF): Every time you eat, a certain percentage of the calories ingested are "burned off" just to digest the food itself. What you eat matters here as some macros are more metabolically demanding to digest.

- Carbohydrates: 5 to 15% of the energy consumed

- Protein: 20 to 35%

- Fats: at most 5 to 15 %

Resting Metabolic Rate (RMR) : RMR is the number of calories you burn each day at rest, just to breathe, think, and live.

Non-Exercise Activity Thermogenesis (NEAT): NEAT is the calories you burn through fidgeting, standing, walking and all other physical activities except purposeful exercise.

So, a number of factors are working against you when trying to lose weight... So what can you do if more exercise and less food isn't really the answer forever?

1. **Eat more protein**

Protein is essential when losing fat.

Protein helps you keep that all-important lean body mass so you don't look like a bag of milk when you've got to your goal weight.

When you're in a significant calorie deficit (i.e. eating less than you burn), your body is happy to feast on muscle for energy. It doesn't tend to throw out just fat and keep muscle... unless you eat lots of protein.

That's why scale weight is not the only measurement of success.

Your diet sucks if it drops as much muscle as it does fat.

How much protein then?

T-Nation reported on a study conducted by Dr. Joey Antonio on 48 bodybuilders. Each of them reported having taken in about 2 g of protein per kilogram every day for the last few years. Dr. Antonio split the group in two. The first group stayed on the same protein intake (NP). The second increased their daily protein intake to 3.4 g per kilogram per day. All of them did the same training program.

The Results

Both groups, the 2.3 g "low" protein group and the 3.4 g high protein group, gained the same amount of muscle. **However, the really high protein group lost much more fat mass, even though they were taking in about 400 more calories a day.** The NP group lost an average 0.3 kg of fat, but the HP group, despite the extra calories, lost an average of 1.6 kg of fat. Percent body fat decreased, too. The percent body fat decrease was -2.4% in the HP group and -0.6% in the NP group.

How could this happen? Dr. Antonio's group speculated that it might have something to do with the thermic effect of protein or TEF as mentioned previously.

Regardless, the study had three main findings:

- Protein overfeeding is unlikely to cause any gains in body fat, and appears to actually reduce body fat.

- It's wrong to conclude that eating anything more than 1.5 to 2.0 g per kilogram of protein is a waste of time.

- Blood tests confirmed that a high-protein intake had no detrimental effects to the kidneys or any other parameters of health.

My suggestion for most is to aim for 1 gram per lb of bodyweight (and sometimes more, as I'll outline later)

One study showed that 40 grams of protein-induced greater muscle protein synthesis than 20 grams in both high and low LBM groups, contradicting previous studies suggesting that MPS after exercise is maximized after ingesting 20–25 grams of high-quality protein.

Overall, a 40-gram dose of whey protein isolate taken immediately after training stimulated MPS to a greater extent than a 20-gram dose.

Take home: Just by eating more protein you burn more calories, because of the increased thermic effect of eating. If you eat 100 calories of protein, you'll only use about 70 calories of it. (remember that embarrassing episode of "meat sweats" at the Brazilian BBQ joint? Yeah, embrace the pit stains.)

2. **Build more muscle**

Your body burns more calories maintaining muscle tissue than it does fat tissue.

How much though?

Some experts estimate that each extra pound of muscle you gain burns 30-50 extra calories a day, while others estimate that a pound of muscle burns 6 calories at rest, compared to 2 calories burned by a pound of fat. It's not a perfect science, and not a huge difference, but it can add up.

I believe there's more to the story here though.

The more muscle, the more storage capacity for glycogen (stored carbohydrates in your muscle cells).

The more muscle, the more insulin sensitive you are.

The more muscle, the better your body performs.

Take home: Do everything you can to build and maintain every ounce of lean muscle.

Footnote: Muscle isn't just for looking good. Artero, et al., (2012) did a review of the literature on the effects of increased muscle strength and found that it has a protective effect on all-cause and cancer mortality in healthy middle-aged men, men with high blood pressure, and those with existing heart disease.

3. **Eat every damn macronutrient (within reason)**

A balanced diet is sustainable.

A balanced diet will over the long haul.

As mentioned, **protein should form the base of your fat loss diet.**

Aim for 1-1.5g per lb of bodyweight, particularly if you exercise regularly and want to maintain or gain some muscle along the way (and who doesn't ... seriously).

Then utilize carbs in moderation – enough to fuel training, boost leptin (maintains metabolism), and promotes happy chemicals in your brain. Have you gone zero carb? Yeah, you were an asshole every minute of that diet, right? No need to drop carbs to zero and hate life. From the Department of Captain Obvious, in addition to starchy and fruit carbs, get in some greens. Vegetables are loaded with vitamins, minerals, and fibre to help you fill up during meals without the calorie cost.

Then comes fats. Fats are tricky. A lot of fad diets and fitness influencers would like you to believe you can defy the laws of physics (Energy Balance Equation) and somehow lose weight in a significant calorie surplus through eating fats and keeping carbs on the sidelines.

Fats are fine – in moderation – but there's no magic there, no matter what some guru tells you. You don't need heaps of butter and coconut oil in your coffee to get your brain working in the morning. One little tablespoon of butter has as many calories as almost a pound-and-a-half of fresh spinach.

Fats keep your sex hormones healthy, boost the immune system, and are satiating, but very calorie dense and blow up a diet if you aren't careful. Stick to tight portion control.

Peanut butter on toast, these photos look nearly identical but the one on the left has 10g of peanut butter and the one on the right has 50g of peanut butter.

A subtle difference which equates to 260 more calories. Very easy to do on calorie-dense fats like oils, spreads and nut butter.

As much as you may hate to hear it, if you are struggling to manage your weight it is quite possible that your guesswork sucks.

Take home: Eat a balance of all three macronutrients, proteins, fats and carbs, then add in veggies, but pay particular attention to your portions.

4. Adjust course when you hit a sticking point

As your weight loss progresses, the plan that got you from A to B may not get you to C.

Small adjustments can add up here.

Maybe it's removing 5-10% of your calories from carbs and fats.

Maybe it's adding in an extra walk or two each week.

Maybe it's upping your workout volume in the gym by small increments.

However, one study referenced on Precision Nutrition found weight loss plateaus have less to do with metabolic adaptations and more to do with "an intermittent lack of diet adherence" – i.e. in scientific terms, eating too much shit too often.

Take home: Do an objective review of your actual diet in relation to your expenditure or hire a third party coach to help you get out of your own way.

5. Cut back on processed foods

This transitions nicely from my last point. Stop eating so much shit foods, you're a grown adult! If it comes in a box and has a long list of ingredients, avoid it for the most part.

For a number of reasons, **the first of which is we absorb more calories from highly processed carbohydrates and fats, because they're easier to digest.**

For example, research found that almost 38 percent of the fat in peanuts was excreted in the stool, rather than absorbed by the body. Whereas seemingly all of the fat in peanut butter was absorbed. Whole foods are more complete (with lots of fibre for one) and harder to digest as a result.

There are two problems with eating junk food.

The first: Your brain is doing its job to keep you alive. Junk food is full of calories and highly palatable. Your brain knows it should load up on these calories while it can, in the event of famine down the road. Remember, your brain was programmed during a time when food was scarce or hard to come by.

The second: Junk foods also give us a "hit" or a reward. We'll go out of our way to get foods with a high reward value. Do you stand in line at Starbucks? Busted.

Take home: Eat more whole, fresh, minimally processed foods with a balance of macronutrients, protein, carbs and fats. Keep the junk out of sight. It's the only way to minimize temptations.

6. **Have patience**

Motivation wanes. You need daily, consistent effort and habits to succeed over the long haul.

That means you're going to have to view your weight loss journey as a marathon, not a sprint.

Smart weight loss can and should be relatively slow, as most recommendations suggest you aim to lose about 0.5-1 percent of your body weight per week.

This slow and steady approach helps to maintain muscle mass and minimize the adaptive metabolic responses to a lower calorie intake and resulting weight loss. Faster weight loss tends to result in more muscle loss without extra fat loss, as well as a larger adaptive response.

7. **Do the right amount of exercise FOR YOU**

Resistance training is the Big Kahuna. Training helps you maintain muscle in a calorie deficit, according to lots of studies I'm failing to mention here.

When dieting, you'll need to do a bit more exercise than you were doing to maintain your weight.

But make small changes at first.

I suggest you add in metabolic resistance training. It increases the metabolic cost of exercise through post-exercise oxygen consumption (EPOC). The more you can create a deficit through exercise, the better, as it means you don't have to drop your food intake even lower.

But don't overdo it. How much is too much? That depends on you, as everyone's recovery abilities vary based on lifestyle, genetics and a host of other factors.

One way to increase your training "tolerance" is active recovery work (e.g. meditation, walking). These low-intensity activities help you balance your training and lifestyle by decreasing stress (lowering cortisol).

My quick tip for the busy person is to take a 10-minute cool down walk or lay down on a mat with relaxing music in your earbuds after every strength training workout. Easy, right?

8. **Find ways to increase NEAT.**

Remember NEAT mentioned earlier in this novel of a post?

As you diet down, you'll find yourself uncontrollably beckoned to Netflix and the couch.

This is your body's attempt to down-regulate NEAT now that is has fewer calories to work with.

It largely happens without you realizing it, so you need to set some rules to keep yourself active.

Take the stairs. Park further away. Use a step counter and set a daily target.

These small increases in activity can make a big difference.

Take home: Do less sitting, more moving. The lower you take your calories, the more likely your body will down-regulate activity. You'll need to schedule in activity to make it happen, even when the couch and Netflix beckon.

To recap, 8 ways to diet down beyond just more exercise:

1. Eat lots of protein

2. Build more muscle

3. Eat every macronutrient (in moderation)

4. Adjust course when you plateau

5. Cut back on processed foods

6. Have patience

7. Do the right amount of exercise for you

8. Find ways to increase NEAT

The Biggest Losers ended up bigger than they started.

According to a study published in the journal *Obesity*, only one of the 14 Biggest Loser contestants studied weighs less today than when the competition wrapped.

The culprit appears to be the contestants' metabolisms, which slowed down as they lost weight rapidly for the show, according to the research presented.

How can you avoid the mistakes of Biggest Loser contestants, stare a big weight loss goal in the face and come out the other side at a sustainable weight?

Well, for one, most weight-loss programs recommend that people lose about one to two pounds per week.

One reason for that, apart from keeping metabolism operational, is people who lose weight fast have a greater loss of muscle than those who lose weight at a more moderate pace. The plan enclosed in this book will guide you.

The Law of Red Velvet Cake

Red Velvet Cake...

My guilty pleasure.

Specifically, the one a local iconic restaurant, Salisbury House, makes...

The icing.. to die for.

The melt in your mouth filling... orgasmic.

But *The Law of Red Velvet Cake* keeps me honest.

It goes like this:

If the cake doesn't get into my car, it doesn't get home.

And if it doesn't get home, it doesn't get in my mouth.

And if it doesn't get in my mouth, it doesn't contribute to belly fat.

You feel me?

If the temptation is in the house, you are going to indulge eventually.

This rule can be applied to your guilty pleasure.

What is it you can't help yourself around?

Make sure it isn't staring at you from the pantry.

PS. When you are ready, here are the 3 best ways I can help you transform your Dad Bod into a superhero physique.

Chapter 2

Eating like a man

Why you need red meat

By now you've probably heard of the Netflix documentary What the Health, the movie that looks to convince you there's only one way to eat for overall health – going vegan.

What The Health, like many documentaries that came before it, does make some truthful points, but offers a narrow view of the science with cherry-picked studies to support the views of filmmaker Kip Anderson, who is not a scientist. But he did seek out a slew of vegan-friendly health professionals to reinforce the film's claims.

Of course, there's no doubt we are in the midst of a health epidemic. As men, we have never been fatter and lacking in testosterone. And, yes, most of us could stand to eat more fruits and vegetables and less processed meat and dairy. But scare tactics documentaries like this portray do more harm than good.

Let's look at the facts:

A Calorie Deficit Matters Most

First, if you're overeating and sedentary, no diet will save you.

If you're overweight, focus on losing weight first and foremost, and that starts and ends with eating less than you need to maintain your body weight.

Case in point: Mark Haub, a professor of nutrition at Kansas State University, proved that calories-in versus calories-out is what matters first when seeking weight loss. Haub limited himself to 1,800 calories a day, eating Twinkies or another treat every three hours instead of actual meals, while also consuming a protein shake and some vegetables over the course of the diet.

Haub not only lost weight but improved all biomarkers of health along with it. His LDL, considered the bad cholesterol, decreased, while his HDL, or good cholesterol, increased by 30%. And he reduced his triglycerides by 39%.

Need a place to start? Grab this free Mansformation Cheat Sheet that includes a nutrition plan (yes, it recommends red meat).

Will Bacon Kill You?

Know this: Eating bacon on Saturday mornings will not cause you to instantly drop dead, face down in your frying pan.

The dose makes the poison.

If you make a habit of eating bacon for breakfast, chargrilled BBQ hot dogs for lunch, and processed deli meats for dinner, day in and out, yes, you may, in fact, be increasing your risk for colorectal cancer. But regularly swapping those processed meats for grass-fed beef, wild caught fish and lean chicken is a completely different story.

It's the processed kind that are more likely to cause colorectal cancer, according to the World Health Organization's 2015 review of the link between processed meat and cancer. What The Health conveniently ignores this fact.

You'd be doing yourself a disservice by eliminating red meat entirely – it's one of the most nutrient-dense foods out there (organ meats like liver are even better), packed full of fat soluble vitamins and protein to positively impact your hormonal profile (think testosterone), build muscle and boost mental clarity.

Red meat supplies vitamin B12, which helps DNA synthesis and keeps nerve and red blood cells healthy, and zinc, which keeps the immune system working properly, as well as protein to build and repair muscle.

Further still, a meta-analysis, reported on by Examine.com, based on 24 randomized controlled trials in adults, compared red meat eaters to those who didn't consume red meat. Compared with eating less than an ounce of red meat per day, consuming more meat does not appear to have a significant influence on blood cholesterol, triglycerides, or blood pressure, according to the research.

The study also noted that red meat is likely to be more harmful when prepared in certain ways. Harsher cooking methods such as frying, broiling, BBQ grilling, and roasting consistently led to higher levels of toxic compounds than gentler cooking methods such as boiling, poaching, stewing, and steaming.

It would be quite the stretch to state that a charbroiled burger patty, bacon or sausage are the same as a medium-rare sirloin steak or ground grass-fed beef.

Is Eating Eggs Every Day As Bad As Smoking Five Cigarettes?

This other claim from WTH reflects an out-of-date understanding of cholesterol's role in health. According to Vox.com, two in three long-term smokers will die as a result of their habit. The same just isn't true for egg eaters.

Cholesterol was wrongly considered a scapegoat for decades, and the scientific community has moved on since evidence has piled up showing that eating more cholesterol isn't necessarily associated with higher levels in the blood or an increased risk of heart disease. That's why it's been declassified as a "nutrient of concern" in the American diet.

What Everyone Can Agree On

There is no best diet universally. You need to determine the diet best suited to you. The nutrition community has generally moved away from prescribing particular diets or vilifying foods.

For example, a recent consensus statement reported on by Vox. com from a diverse group of nutrition researchers came to these conclusions:

A healthy dietary pattern is higher in vegetables, fruits, whole grains, low- or non-fat dairy, seafood, legumes, and nuts; moderate in alcohol (among adults); lower in red and processed meats; and low in sugar-sweetened foods and drinks and refined grains.

Additional strong evidence shows that it is not necessary to eliminate food groups or conform to a single dietary pattern to achieve healthy dietary patterns. Rather, individuals can combine foods in a variety of flexible ways to achieve healthy dietary patterns, and these strategies should be tailored to meet the individual's health needs, dietary preferences and cultural traditions.

There's a lot of evidence that plant-based diets can be a truly effective strategy for many people. Also, there's the whole animal rights movement to veganism, which is a valid reason to switch.

But when it comes to dieting for weight loss or general health, there is simply no one-size-fits-all solution. Anyone who tells you otherwise is trying to sell you something or blind to the facts.

Raise Your T Like Mr. T

Here's one area I always see overlooked by clients.

Getting your hormones right.

Particularly your thyroid and sex hormones. A standard blood test will show you where you stand, but even if you're in the "healthy" range as defined by the medical community, you may not be optimal (for fat loss, energy, mood & ALL of the above)

Here are my top 12 (or so – didn't count) ways to boost your testosterone. I'll be back with a thyroid blog post later this week, but that one's trickier. Both of these hormones are present in women and should be prioritized (not just men).

Sleep.

I've got bad news for all you night owls: testosterone is directly related to the amount of sleep you get each night. The more sleep, the more you increase your testosterone. Sleep also boosts Growth Hormone and rebuilds your brain. Want an easy way to increase your testosterone? Turn off the TV and computer and go to bed!

Weight Lifting.

Scientists aren't really sure how it raises testosterone, but then does it really matter? The important thing is that pumping iron pumps up your baseline testosterone by about 15% according to one study referenced in Lee Myers *Natural vs. Testosterone Therapy*. Though other studies have suggested the opposite (my hunch is only when nutrition does not allow for proper recovery, spiking cortisol levels. High testosterone can't live in unison with high cortisol)

Attitude.

Your outlook on life controls just about everything, so why not your testosterone as well? Depression will destroy your testosterone and the opposite will increase your testosterone. In other words, it's not just your huevos that pump out an increase in testosterone, it's that head of yours.

Competition.

Play a sport? Beer league? Same deal. Even the anticipation of competition can significantly boost testosterone in men. Having a little healthy competition in your life is a GOOD thing.

Watch the Sugar.

According to another study in Lee Myer's work: blood sugar spikes lead to decreased testosterone. In fact, blood sugar elevation can whack testosterone by as much as 25%! Furthermore, it does not matter whether you are diabetic, pre-diabetic or normal: your testosterone will suffer just the same.

In fact, it actually drove testosterone so low that a significant number of the men became hypogonadal during the test! And the researchers found that this was not just a transient result: testosterone was still significantly lowered two hours after the test. This is yet another example of the importance of watching your Glycemic Load and managing your blood sugar levels.

Metabolic Syndrome.

Metabolic Syndrome (prediabetes or Met-S) is associated with lower levels of testosterone [source], and most Americans over 40 or so have a full-blown case of it. In fact, researchers have concluded that "while it is clear that the metabolic syndrome can suppress circulating testosterone levels, it has also been documented that low testosterone levels induce the metabolic syndrome ".

Stress

You think you thrive on stress. And to a degree, a moderate dose of stress is good for you. Adrenaline is a "rush" after all, right? What we don't realize is that not all our hormones, such as adrenaline and cortisol, go up with stress. Some hormones, your beloved testosterone in particular, head south very quickly under those conditions. In fact, what science has found is that if your cortisol, the primary stress hormone, is high enough, it is the culprit in shutting down testosterone directly.

Alcohol

Heavy alcohol consumption can lead to zinc depletion, which in turn can lead to lower testosterone levels. A pint on a Friday or Saturday night? All good. But drinking more than two drinks (for men) daily is considered heavy consumption. One binge can do your T in.

Drop the Extra Weight.

There is nothing uglier than those love handles to your health: they are estrogen factories. Fat converts ever increasing amounts of your precious testosterone into estradiol, the chief estrogen. As a verification, low testosterone is correlated to being overweight. Myers also mentioned a study that examined 64 severely obese men: their average testosterone was a measly 340 even though the average age was in the late forties. The same study noted that weight was associated with increased estradiol and decreased testosterone. The authors found that bypass surgery decreased estrogen and increased testosterone significantly! What is interesting is that being overweight lowers SHBG levels, the protein that binds to testosterone, which should translate to higher free testosterone levels. However, multiple studies have shown that being overweight lowers free testosterone as well. So, basically, being overweight does everything negative possible to your hormone levels!

Get Your Thyroid Checked

Hypothyroidism is associated with low testosterone levels. Furthermore, an underactive thyroid has many overlapping symptoms with low testosterone which as mental fog, anxiety, low energy, low libido and the like. This is definitely worth checking if you are struggling with low testosterone. (This can also be a definite issue with Female Libido as well.)

Vitamin D.

Turns out a few cents a day of this all-important vitamin could boost your testosterone levels. Vitamin D is critical for fertility, muscle growth, exercise performance and hundreds of other physiological processes. Correcting a vitamin D deficiency, which is quite common, can lead to a bump in total testosterone of about 30% according to a number of studies. Warning: Calcium supplementation has recently been shown to decrease Vit D absorption, so get your calcium from food. If you don't want to pop a supplement, get 10 minutes of midday sun exposure in the summer (3-4 times per week).

Suggest finding a combination vitamin D3/vitamin K2. Vitamin D provides improved bone development by helping you *absorb* calcium, but there is new evidence that vitamin K2 *directs the calcium* to your skeleton, while preventing it from being deposited where you don't want it, in your arteries. A large part of arterial plaque consists of calcium deposits (atherosclerosis), hence the term "hardening of the arteries."

Magnesium.

What dirt cheap supplement might give you a nice boost in testosterone, according to a recent study? Magnesium is very inexpensive and was found in a study of seniors to be tightly correlated with T levels. And it is no wonder: magnesium is used by literally hundreds of critical systems in the body. Another very interesting study noted that magnesium levels increased testosterone when combined with exercise.

I recommend magnesium citrate, not magnesium oxide. The latter is more of a laxative. Take this an hour or so before bed, not in the AM or it'll affect your wakefulness!

Spare Tire. Beer Belly.

It doesn't matter what you call it, those extra pounds around your middle have been correlated with lower testosterone. Furthermore, studies have shown that giving men testosterone will decrease visceral fat a little. The reverse is also likely true: the more visceral fat that you accumulate, the lower your testosterone levels.

Content for this chapter provided by Natural vs. Testosterone Therapy by Lee Myers. The medical and/or nutritional information is not intended to be a substitute for professional medical advice, diagnosis, or treatment. Always seek the advice of your physician or other qualified health provider with any questions you may have regarding a medical condition. Never disregard professional medical advice or delay seeking it because of something you have read here.

The Cinderella Diet

Heard of The Cinderella Diet?

You may have seen the news reports on this...

Currently trending in Japan, the practice of calculating one's "Cinderella weight" has been gaining traction.

A diet in which the end goal is to have similar proportions to Cinderella—you know, that fictional, petite Disney character with a waist the size of a stick.

One calculates their "goal" Cinderella weight by squaring one's height in meters, then multiplying that number by 18.

A few (major) problems with this

Some (most) people have no business trying to achieve a BMI of 18.

We all have different bone structures and genetic blueprints.

For myself, I have wide hips. When I'm ultra lean, they're still wide but no longer padded and they dig into my wife during cuddle time (sorry, hun)

I'm built to be a bigger guy. Doesn't mean I can't get my bodyfat fairly low, but trying to have the beach body male model look is a LOSING battle.

Past attempts to get there meant extreme mood swings and a lot of daytime lethargy, not conducive to being a parent with two careers.

For women, extreme dieting can have unwanted side effects such as tanked energy levels and even irregular or full-blown loss of periods in extreme cases.

So, by all means, have goals...

But, remember, even after getting lean, that person staring back at you in the mirror is just going to be a smaller version of the person you see today - with the same curves, 'flaws' and strengths.

Cheat on your diet more

After a holiday season full of overindulgence, you are particularly motivated (or guilty) to start a healthy lifestyle this time of year.

Regardless of all that enthusiasm, most New Year's resolutions fall off by mid-February.

The statistics are grim – with some dudes in lab coats who did a study claiming only 8% achieve their goals.

That's not surprising – especially when you consider most go to extremes trying to undo the holidays with a diet comprised of nothing but celery sticks and tears.

How can you change your success rate this year? Cheat on your diet more.

Say what?

According to Australian researchers (thanks, guys!) a group taking frequent diet breaks lost ~50% more fat compared to a group dieting continuously for 16 weeks.

The researchers recruited 51 obese men and divided them into two groups.

All were put on a diet geared toward weight loss, providing only 67% of the calories needed to maintain their weight.

The first group was the control group who dieted for 16 consecutive weeks.

The second group undertook a 30-week diet, alternating two weeks of dieting with two weeks of maintenance calories throughout.

The Results

Aside from losing 50% more fat overall, almost all of the extra pounds of weight lost by the diet break group was fat as well.

But the positive results didn't end there. The researchers continued to monitor both groups for a period of six months after the study's conclusion.

Both regained some weight, but weight loss in the diet break group was 17.9 pounds greater than the control group overall.

One caveat: The diet break group did take twice as long to accomplish their results (30 weeks compared to 16) but the researchers believed the breaks helped prevent the slowing of one's metabolism, a common side effect of aggressive diets over the long haul.

Also of equal importance is the fact these diet breaks weren't a two-week bender filled with Chinese buffets. The men still tracked their calories, with a return to 'maintenance' calories 33% higher than on the diet, while still keeping tabs on weight gain. During these diet breaks in the study, there was no loss or gain of body weight. I.E. They didn't go off the rails.

BONUS: Grab this free Mansformation diet cheat sheet and get a simple and sustainable nutrition plan to help drop those first 10 or so pounds. Warning: You might need to create a new hole in your belt as your waist shrinks.

More Proof Diet Breaks Can Work...

In another study, scientists from the University of Quebec put 15 gym rats (all men) on a "Super Size Me" diet, comprised of nothing but McDonald's for two weeks.

Breakfast, lunch and dinner filled with nothing but Egg McMuffins, Big Macs, fries and coke (yes, they even ditched the diet coke!).

Sounds like some sort of twisted heaven for the fat kid inside you, right?

Throughout the short study, they also did daily 30-minute high-intensity interval sessions on a treadmill, sprinting full out followed by a recovery time, rinse and repeat.

Surely, despite the cardio, their insides were rotting and the scale ballooned?

Wrong.

They didn't gain weight.

And their health, according to the researchers, improved aside from a negative drop in HDL cholesterol (considered the 'good' cholesterol).

Of course, this study was only two weeks long. Had they continued to eat this way, you'd have to assume things may turn for the worse.

You know how you feel when you supply your body with a quality, balanced diet full of micronutrients, not junk food. It just works better, right?

Plus, who can expect to "out-train" a bad diet with DAILY HIIT sessions? You're asking to hit a wall eventually.

But, the good news is if you're feeling guilty about a holiday binge or two – don't sweat it. Just brush it off and get back on plan. The impact of a bad day of diet isn't nearly as damaging as you think.

Frankly, clients often fret a vacation away. When they return and they get back to their structured diet regimen and back to checking in with me again, they often report being "shocked" at how fast their weight returned to pre-vacation levels, something that has never happened before.

How Can You Apply This?

Unless you have a pressing weight loss goal like an upcoming vacation, wedding or bodybuilding show, you can take the long view and mix in short-term periods of diet breaks like the two above examples and do just fine over the long haul.

However, you could theoretically take less frequent breaks, and achieve similar (or better) results in less time.

As you know, if your diet is filled with restrictions, as soon as you return to old habits, the weight creeps back on.

One way around that just might be built-in diet breaks, so you have something to look forward to throughout the process.

How Stosh Got Swole

Stosh was your typical dad.

A business owner with 2 kids and a full life.

All the pieces were there. But one day, in late 2014, he realized one important element was being neglected: his own health.

60 pounds overweight, he decided to go all in on losing the weight, and that he did, dropping 80 pounds.

Fast forward to 2017 and he had largely kept the weight off, but something just wasn't right.

"I realized I hardly had any muscle mass. I kinda had chicken wings," Stosh said. "But I struggled with all of the conflicting advice you read about online about weightlifting and your diet."

That's when Stosh reached out, becoming one of the Mansformers in my coaching program

"I've been friends with Mitch on Facebook for a few years and I noticed I really found his daily tips and strategies he would post helpful, so I contacted him for some advice and he pointed me in the direction of his Mansformers program.

"I decided to join because I was tired of the B.S. online and I'm the kind of person who works better when I'm held accountable for something and when I have someone to make me accountable for the work I do.

"Mitch is good at what he does and clearly loves what he does and this integrity shines through in his program," Stosh adds.

"After 5 months, my body fat percentage has never been lower and my muscle mass has never been higher and my general and mental health have also never been better."

"I would and will recommend this program to anyone who is, like me, an amateur who needs professional help looking to improve their overall health," Stosh says. "Because that's exactly what I received, professional, fun help to get me into the best shape of my life."

Frankly, Stosh was that dream client who takes direction, asks questions when he's not sure about something and then does the work.

It's also a bonus that he's from Northwestern Ontario just a stone's throw from my birthplace of Eagle River. I also worked at the restaurant he now owns back in the summers during high school... small world.

Stosh just graduated the program with honours. (If I was to give out such elitist pieces of paper, anyway).

FREE Download: Have a fair bit of fat to lose, especially in the belly? Need a place to start in 30 seconds or less? Grab this easily digestible (pun intended) two-page cheat sheet for men, to simplify your diet without fads, quick fixes or calorie counting, courtesy of coach Mitch.

Chapter 3

You're an addict, man (but so am I)

Your brain loves Big Macs

What is about chocolate, pizza, Big Macs and sweets that make it so hard to stop at "just one"?

You know these foods aren't good for you in excess, so why do you indulge?

Is it the forbidden fruit mentality? You want what you can't have?

For starters, your brain loves junk food.

Junk foods are energy dense (i.e. high in calories). Good news if you're a hunter-gatherer and nutrients are scarce, but bad news in today's society of endless food at your fingertips.

But what's happening inside your brain that drives this response?

Stephan Guyenet referenced several studies in an article on Examine. com, which show your mouth and small intestine detect the base materials in sugar, fat, and protein and send a signal to the brain that releases dopamine.

And the more concentrated the nutrients (think junk food) the greater the surge in dopamine.

Essentially, your brain is doing its job by encouraging you to pursue calorie dense foods that would help your distant ancestors stay alive or survive periods of famine. But your brain chemistry simply wasn't built for the world you live in today.

You need simply take a passing glance at that timely pizza promotion in your mailbox and crave it because the sensory cues are so innate. Then, with a few clicks on your smartphone, that cheesy delight arrives at your doorstep.

How can you avoid these temptations? Plan ahead. Prepare wholesome meals to bring to work with you so you aren't starving and accidentally on purpose reach for that doughnut in the lunchroom. Download this handy "Mansformation Cheat Sheet" to set yourself up with a nutrition plan for success. I.E. Opt for a filling quinoa salad with a variety of nutrients over a Unicorn Frap from Starbucks.

Drug-Like Effects

Further still, some junk foods combine calories with drug-like effects.

Guyenet writes about chocolate's mix of calories and a drug called theobromine. Much like its cousin caffeine, theobromine is a mild stimulant. This drug accentuates fat and sugar's natural ability to spike dopamine signalling, which in many people results in powerful cravings and addictive-like behaviour.

Do you remember the first time you drank coffee or beer? You likely didn't love the taste.

But coffee has caffeine and beer has alcohol, two drugs that your brain gets a reward from.

So, in turn, your sensory cues tell you to pay $6 for that Frappuccino and elbow your way through a crowd to get to the bar.

Social Norms

Our society also associates eating with pleasure at every turn.

At the movies, you're expected to get a big popcorn and coke.

You can't watch that ball game without a big bratwurst.

Poker with the guys? Round of drinks and wings for all.

Those are powerful social cues to overcome. But it'll take replacing old habits with new, healthy ones to buck those trends.

Bring a protein bar in your pocket to the theatre.

Eat a filling, healthy dinner before you head to the game.

Set some ground rules for that poker night (like a drink limit).

And, yes, you may have to overcome peer pressure and stick to your guns.

So is it futile to try to attempt another diet?

Not necessarily.

How to re-program your brain:

Eat more whole, fresh, minimally processed foods with a balance of macronutrients, protein, carbs and fats so you aren't "shortchanging" your brain from much-needed nutrients (i.e. limit cravings)

Eat slowly and mindfully. No matter what you eat, slowing down will help your digestive system do its job and also help your brain get the signal from your gut that it's full

Keep temptations out of sight. Easier said than done, but work to control your home environment. Don't buy Costco-sized ice cream or sweets – only indulge in controlled amounts. I.E. Opt for a kid-sized McFlurry on the way home instead of buying a two-gallon pail of ice cream at the store. If tempting, unhealthy foods aren't within arm's reach, not only will they be harder to eat, but you'll be less likely to crave them.

Get this handy "Mansformation Cheat Sheet" cheat sheet to set yourself up with a nutrition plan

Chapter 4

Choose your hard

I wish I knew the source of that quote.

But it's undeniably true.

The easy choice (on the surface) is often harder down the road.

Sure, working out is HARD.

Cutting back on junk food is HARD.

Stopping at two beers is HARD.

Alternatively, sitting on the couch is easy, at least at first.

But being overweight is HARDER.

Taking statins to manage your cholesterol is HARDER.

Not being a good role model for your kids is HARDER.

The advantages to being severely overweight I can count on one hand...

Free burgers at Heart Attack Grill. Check.

Your BMR is higher so you can eat more to maintain your weight. Check.

...Anything else?

So, if most things in life are hard regardless, why not choose a "hard" that's in your control?

Trading an hour of gym time for 24 hours of discomfort makes sense to me.

Choose your hard.

Red Bull and vodka, lost pants and lessons learned

Trying to get in shape without clear direction is like canoeing upstream without a paddle.

You've probably seen Elliptical Lady and Ab Machine Man at your local gym.

These two seemingly live at the gym, but they have no clearly defined goals or a clear plan of attack – they're simply going through the motions – and look exactly the same year after year.

There needs to be a plan of action in place.

Elliptical Lady's body can do that 30-minute cardio routine in its sleep, so expecting to improve conditioning or drop fat from it is wishful thinking at this stage. She's gotten all the benefits out of that.

Maybe you've taken the first step and purchased a gym membership before (or currently have one that's only serving to auto-debit monthly from your chequing account).

Maybe you gave it an honest effort as part of your New Year's Resolution one time, but didn't see the results fast enough and gave up.

Maybe you are working hard right now, but need to work smarter to accelerate your progress.

Hell, when I was a cardio bunny running miles every day I was working harder than I am now, but my look and how I feel is far superior today.

20 minutes a day gets you started – strategic planning and pushing outside your comfort zone makes it lasting.

We are all creatures of habit. But why dedicate an hour to the gym every day if it's not going to physically change you or improve conditioning, muscle gains etc. (whatever your goal is)?

You need to find the minimum effective dose of exercise (and eating right) that gets results and allows you to still live the lifestyle you want.

Anyway, let me tell you a story...

I used to be the most vanilla dude ever in high school (closely related to my weight and lack of confidence).

I was more focused on playing video games and hitting on cyber gaming girls (well, at least I hope they were girls) than getting out and socializing.

I sacrificed growing as an individual and building friendships during those formative years, and had to play catch-up in my 20s.

But once I started to get in shape and ended up in a university setting, rather than take the balanced approach, I did a complete 180.

I wanted so badly to fit in that I went full Party Boy from Jackass mode. (See what I mean in this <u>video</u>)

My first night out with my new college crew ended up being sloppy.

Here's how it went down... (sorry, Mom)

I guzzled one too many Red Bull & vodkas pre-gaming,

Allegedly tried to pull the top down of a female classmate while at the club (I say allegedly because I don't remember this, but it haunted me for several years after),

Puked in a cab and got momentarily chased by said cabbie, but thankfully he didn't want to abandon his car and gave up quickly (my "run" was more of a stagger),

Got picked up by a RANDOM car full of teenagers/young adults who found my state of inebriation VERY amusing (I still can't picture their faces, but do remember their laughter),

Managed to get dropped off on the right street by slurring the name of it repeatedly, but instead of going straight home, I jumped a fence and ripped my pants (abandoning them there on the spot),

Mercifully, I eventually awoke on the couch to the disapproval of my parents (it was Remembrance Day – my way of honouring our troops was to not remember much of the night before).

As the cherry on the gong show sundae, this was winter and it was very cold here in Canada. Pants not optional in other words.

Anyway, WTF is this trying to tell you?

Find the balance!

The example above is life-focused, but the same goes for your fitness pursuits.

If you go full bore with monk-like discipline with your eating and training, eventually you're going to burn out or fall off the wagon.

But, alternatively, a directionless approach to fitness "when you get around to it" serves no purpose either.

Moderation doesn't have to mean half-assed. Kill it in the gym, eat right for your body type (most of the time) and then live your life the other 23 hours of the day.

Chapter 5

Putting It All Together

Shed stubborn belly fat

You've been told spot reduction is impossible.

You laugh at the ladies (and some men) wearing their 'waist trimmers' (don't stop laughing at them)

And you think to yourself "Just eat clean and train hard."

Right?

Sure. That's all I knew for the better part of a decade.

You know these things too... but that doesn't mean they help you do them consistently.

(Stay with me here... it'll all make sense very soon).

I lived like a monk in pursuit of the perfect body for years.

I watched everything I put in my mouth and sacrificed a lot.

I would never eat the foods I loved — and never dared miss a meal for fear of losing 'muscle'

On top of that, I trained excessively as often as I could.

Did it work?

Sure, well, maybe, but I could've gotten there an easier way.

Let me explain...

These days, I don't spend hours in the gym. I'm building a business, have a beautiful family and work with a growing roster of guys across the globe.

I eat fun 'off limit' food such as hamburgers and fries, ice cream and guess what?

I found a way to look decent and feel great anyway.

My bloodwork is top shelf, according to my doc.

Plus, I enjoy the process a lot more these days.

The diet isn't a chore because I always have something to look forward to.

The workouts are of my choosing, not some random roided up bodybuilder.

I THOUGHT I had to eat dry chicken every day.

I THOUGHT I had to do crazy workouts, buy a ton of supplements and wash it down with a fancy shake immediately after.

But I now realize this is unsustainable when you have other priorities in your life.

And all of my clients are in the same boat.

But we know there's a fine line there. You are reading this book for a reason. You are not your average Dad Bod totin', lethargic couch potato.

It's no different in the gym.

As a guy, you've probably dealt with stubborn belly fat at one time or another...

The Belly Fat Solution

Now, according to science, you can actually spot target that stubborn stuff – with the right approach to training.

Poor blood flow to certain areas of the body – obliques and lower abs for example – equates to poor fat loss from those areas. Hence the 'stubborn' term.

But the right training strategy can shift calorie burning toward localized areas of fat storage. (Stallknecht, 2007)

Blood flow and lipolysis (i.e. fat burning) are generally higher in subcutaneous adipose tissue adjacent to the contracting muscle.

In layman's terms, if you train your abs the right way at the right time, the belly fat on the outside of the abs will "burn" preferentially when you throw some conditioning work at it.

Essentially, finish your workout going back and forth between an ab exercise and a conditioning exercise.

Pick an ab exercise. Any movement will work. The goal is just to direct blood flow toward that area. For maximum effect, you want the ab set to last 45-60 seconds. Less than that and you won't be getting as much blood flow to the region, according to an article on T-Nation.

Then jump to a conditioning exercise. Any demanding energy systems activity will work here. Sprints, hill sprints, Prowler pushing, battle ropes, tire flipping, etc.

You want the whole session to be non-stop for 10-15 minutes, supersetting the two exercises with minimal rest.

Plan B

In a more recent study, the researchers tested this hypothesis with a small change – pairing steady state cardio (not HIIT) with circuits.

In this study, combining circuit-based resistance training with steady state endurance exercise (i.e. 30 minutes at a steady pace on a bike) resulted in fat mass reduction adjacent to the trained muscle due to enhanced blood flow. In other words, train legs followed by cardio, and your leg bodyfat will reduce preferentially.

One problem: Excessive cardio (or timing cardio and weights concurrently in this fashion) can have an "interference" effect on the muscular adaptations you want to occur after resistance training.

If building muscle is your primary focus, exercise caution with this strategy and/or separate weights and cardio by several hours (or even days).

Now, let's be clear. This is only a couple studies as well. Many other studies stand in contrast, showing localized fat loss adjacent to trained muscles do not occur. No study stands on its own, especially those with small sample sizes.

Further still, spot reduction is not something you need to worry about when you have a lot of body fat to lose all over.

Setting Up The Mansformation Diet

The goal is neither to lose nor gain weight, but rather to add muscle and strength while losing body fat. It's not to say that you won't lose weight or gain weight, but that's not the goal of this program and your bodyweight or scale weight is really an afterthought. The more fat you have to lose, the more likely you can add/maintain muscle while dieting it off – to a point.

The diet during the week is lower carb.

The diets on weekends focus on higher-carb nutrition. You'll also be able to indulge in more social eating (or drinking) on the weekends if you so desire (and of course in moderation).

Please refer to visual guide to determine how to portion your meals appropriately, courtesy of Precision Nutrition's expert guidelines.

Mansformation Diet Plan

Day	Activity Level	Carb Level	Meal Breakdown
Monday	- 30-60 minutes walking - Workout #1	Lower Carb	- 2 Protein/Fat meals - 2 high-protein snacks
Tuesday	- 30-60 minutes walking - Workout #2	Lower Carb	- 2 Protein/Fat meals - 2 high-protein snacks
Wednesday	- 30-60 minutes walking Rest day	Lower Carb	- 2 Protein/Fat meals - 2 high-protein snacks
Thursday	- 30-60 minutes walking Rest day	Lower Carb	- 2 Protein/Fat meals - 2 high-protein snacks
Friday	- 30-60 minutes walking - Workout #3	Higher Carb	- 1 Protein/Carb meal - **1 Fun Meal*** - 2 high-protein snacks
Saturday	- 30-60 minutes walking - Workout #4	Higher Carb	- 1 Protein/Carb meal - **1 Fun Meal*** - 2 high-protein snacks
Sunday	- 30-60 minutes walking - OFF or Active Recovery	Lower Carb	- 2 Protein/Fat meals - 2 high-protein snacks

*A **Fun Meal** is a Protein/Carb meal with a little flexibility in terms of food/carb sources and amounts. Think burger and baked fries.

NOTE: Alcohol is allowed on Friday OR Saturday (not both) at a 3 drink limit. Think low carb beers, champagne (baller) or low carb mixed drinks (i.e. diet and vodka)

Protein/Fat Meal Visual Guide

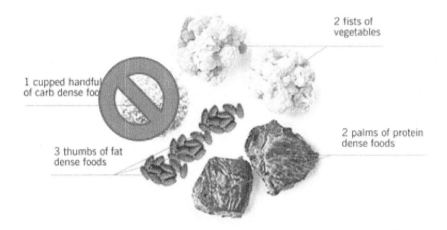

2 fists of
vegetables

1 cupped handful
of carb dense food

2 palms of protein
dense foods

3 thumbs of fat
dense foods

Protein/Carb Meal Visual Guide

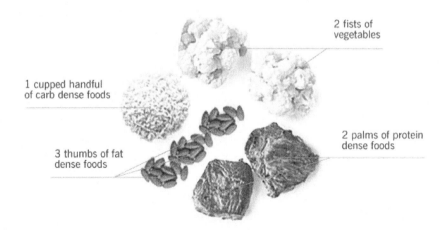

2 fists of
vegetables

1 cupped handful
of carb dense foods

2 palms of protein
dense foods

3 thumbs of fat
dense foods

If you prefer to count calories here's the breakdown:

Bodyweight x 7 on lower carb days

Bodyweight x 12 on higher carb days

I.E. 200 pound man

200 x 7 = 1,400 calories

200 x 12 = 2,400 calories

Get 800 calories from protein (about 200g per day). Fill in the rest with fat/carbs (mostly fat on lower carb days, mostly carbs on higher carb days)

Visual guides brought to you by Precision Nutrition.

What's Next?

Need Mitch's help implementing your Mansformation? Wanna hear more from him? Go to www.mitchcalvert.com.

FREE Download: Have a fair bit of fat to lose, especially in the belly? Need a place to start in 30 seconds or less? Grab this easily digestible (pun intended) two-page <u>cheat sheet</u> for men, to simplify your diet without fads, quick fixes or calorie counting, courtesy of coach Mitch, free for Mansformation Diet readers.

Made in the USA
Coppell, TX
16 June 2023

18172888R10052